Weight Management and Healthy Body Image: Nurturing Your Wellness From Within

permitted by
copyright law.

Table of contents

Chapter 1: The Holistic Approach to Weight Management

Beyond diet and exercise: a comprehensive wellness approach

The role of mental and emotional health in weight management

Long-term vs. short-term goals

Chapter 2: Achieving Sustainable Weight Management

Setting realistic weight management goals

Balancing weight loss with a healthy lifestyle

The importance of
self-compassion and
self-acceptance

Chapter 3: Embracing a Positive Body Image

Understanding body image and its impact on wellness

Strategies for developing a positive body image

Celebrating your unique beauty

Chapter 4: Nutrition and Fitness for Wellness

Science-backed nutrition for weight management

Effective fitness strategies that support both weight management and body confidence

Building a sustainable, balanced routine

Chapter 5: Mindful Wellness

The role of mindfulness and self-care in weight management and body image

Managing stress and building resilience

Cultivating mental and emotional balance

Chapter 6: Building a Supportive Environment

Creating a nurturing and supportive environment for your wellness goals

Seeking social support and understanding

Navigating societal pressures

Introduction

In a world that often fixates on numbers and appearances, it's crucial to recognize that true wellness extends far beyond the scale. The eBook "Weight Management and Healthy Body

Image" delves into a transformative journey where we embrace a holistic approach to well-being, celebrate the significance of cultivating a healthy body image, and provide a comprehensive overview of the eBook's content.

Wellness is a tapestry woven from the threads of physical, emotional, and mental health. It's a harmonious balance that transcends quick fixes and embraces

the long-term
sustainability of a
healthy lifestyle. We
acknowledge that our
journey to wellness
doesn't reside solely
in diet and exercise,
but in fostering a
nurturing relationship
with our bodies,
understanding the
role of mental and

emotional health, and making self-compassion and self-acceptance central to our path.

A healthy body image is a treasure that illuminates our journey. It's the cornerstone of our well-being, empowering us to embrace our unique beauty, nurture self-esteem, and build a loving connection with our bodies. We recognize that, in this pursuit, the scales and mirrors often fall short in reflecting the true essence of our worth. This eBook is a testament to understanding, respecting, and celebrating ourselves for who we truly are.

This comprehensive eBook is your trusted guide on the path to lasting wellness. It will offer a well-rounded exploration of the holistic approach to weight management and nurturing a positive body image. Inside these pages, you'll find:

Strategies for setting realistic, sustainable

weight management goals.

Insights into science-backed nutrition and effective fitness strategies that support your overall well-being.

The powerful role of mindfulness, self-care, and stress

management in your wellness journey.

Guidance on creating a nurturing and supportive environment for your wellness goals.

The art of setting and celebrating milestones that honor your individual journey.

With the holistic approach to wellness, the significance of a healthy body image, and the comprehensive content of this eBook, you're invited to embark on a transformative journey toward a healthier, more body-positive you. It's time to embrace the beauty that lies within, foster a positive connection with your body, and discover the well-being you truly deserve. Let's embark on this transformative journey together.

Chapter 1

The Holistic Approach to Weight Management: Beyond Numbers and Appearance

When we speak of weight management, it's not merely about the numbers on a scale or the superficiality of appearances. This chapter explores the holistic approach to weight management, delving into the importance of looking beyond diet and exercise, recognizing the critical role of mental and emotional health in the journey, and distinguishing between long-term and short-term goals.

Beyond Diet and Exercise: A Comprehensive Wellness Approach

Weight management is a multifaceted endeavor that goes beyond diet and exercise. It's a journey toward comprehensive wellness that encompasses your physical, emotional, and mental health. Here, we embrace a broader perspective that considers not only what you eat and how you move but also how you think, feel, and care for yourself. The holistic approach acknowledges that well-being is a tapestry woven from multiple threads, with

each element playing
a unique and essential
role.

**The Role of Mental
and Emotional Health
in Weight
Management**

Mental and emotional
health are

cornerstones of effective and sustainable weight management. Understanding the emotional triggers behind eating habits, building a positive relationship with food, and managing stress, anxiety, and emotional eating are vital components of a holistic approach. We recognize that a sound mind and emotional balance are prerequisites for achieving your weight management goals.

Long-Term vs. Short-Term Goals

Weight management is often approached with a focus on short-term, immediate results. However, the holistic approach invites us to shift our perspective toward long-term wellness. While short-term goals can be motivating, they should align with a broader, sustainable vision of your health and well-being. This chapter explores the importance of setting realistic long-term goals that prioritize health and self-care over quick fixes.

In adopting the holistic approach to weight management, we recognize that wellness is a journey, not a destination. It's a balanced tapestry of physical, emotional, and mental well-being. As we continue our exploration, we'll delve into the

practical strategies
and insights that can
help you navigate this
journey effectively,
ensuring that your
efforts are aligned
with your long-term
wellness and your
unique vision of a
healthy, happy life.

Chapter 2

Achieving Sustainable Weight Management: Balancing Health and Well-Being

In the pursuit of weight management, sustainability is the key to lasting success. This chapter delves into the components of achieving sustainable weight management, including the importance of setting realistic goals, the balance between weight loss and a healthy lifestyle, and the significance of self-compassion and self-acceptance.

Setting Realistic Weight Management Goals

Your journey toward sustainable weight management begins with setting realistic, achievable goals. While it's natural to aspire to significant changes, it's equally crucial to set objectives that align with your unique circumstances, body, and health. Realistic goals are milestones that are challenging yet attainable, and they provide a path to success. We'll explore strategies for defining these goals in a way that sets you up for success rather than frustration.

Balancing Weight Loss with a Healthy Lifestyle

Sustainable weight management isn't about quick fixes or extreme measures. It's about striking a balance between your weight management objectives and maintaining a healthy, well-rounded lifestyle. We'll discuss the importance of incorporating habits that support overall well-being, such as mindful eating, regular physical activity, and self-care. The chapter emphasizes that true health goes beyond a number on the scale and encourages you

to build a life that
nurtures your body
and mind.

The Importance of Self-Compassion and Self-Acceptance

In your journey to
weight management,
self-compassion and

self-acceptance are your most cherished allies. They guide you through moments of self-doubt and frustration, helping you maintain a positive relationship with yourself and your body. The chapter highlights the power of being kind to yourself, reframing negative self-talk, and embracing your unique beauty and worth.

Achieving sustainable weight management isn't about temporary changes but lifelong well-being. In adopting these principles, you'll navigate your journey with a balanced, positive perspective that prioritizes health, self-care, and self-acceptance. The road to lasting wellness is paved with self-compassion, realistic goals, and a healthy, holistic lifestyle. As we continue to explore the holistic approach to weight management, you'll find practical strategies to apply these principles and foster the well-being you deserve.

Chapter 3

Embracing a Positive Body Image: Celebrating Your Unique Beauty

Our journey toward holistic wellness continues with a deep exploration of body image and its profound impact on our overall well-being. In this chapter, we'll delve into the significance of understanding body image, explore strategies for developing a positive and healthy view of our bodies, and celebrate the unique

beauty that resides
within each of us.

Understanding Body Image and Its Impact on Wellness

Body image refers to
the perceptions,
beliefs, and feelings
we hold about our

bodies. It is a mental and emotional reflection of how we view our physical selves. Our body image can significantly impact our wellness journey. We'll discuss how negative body image can affect our self-esteem, mental health, and

relationships.
Understanding these
influences is a crucial
step in fostering a
healthier, more
positive perspective.

**Strategies for
Developing a Positive
Body Image**

Developing a positive body image is a journey that involves reshaping our beliefs and attitudes. We'll explore a range of strategies that can help us achieve this transformation, including:

**Mindful Self-
Reflection:**
Recognizing and
challenging negative
self-talk and
unrealistic beauty
standards.

**Practicing Self-
Compassion:** Offering
ourselves kindness
and acceptance rather

than criticism and judgment.

Surrounding Ourselves with Positivity: Building a support network that promotes self-esteem and body confidence.

Fostering Gratitude: Embracing gratitude

for our bodies and
their capabilities.

Nurturing Our Bodies:
Engaging in self-care
and self-love practices
that celebrate our
uniqueness.

**Celebrating Your
Unique Beauty**

Every individual possesses a unique beauty that transcends societal standards and expectations. In this section, we'll celebrate this distinctiveness. We'll discuss the importance of acknowledging our beauty beyond physical appearance and valuing our individuality. By recognizing the beauty within, we'll learn to honor our bodies and approach our wellness journey with a more positive and compassionate perspective.

Embracing a positive body image is an integral component of our holistic approach to wellness. By developing a healthier body image and celebrating our unique beauty, we can foster self-esteem, confidence, and well-being that transcends numbers and appearances. This chapter is an invitation to rediscover your beauty from within and begin a transformative journey toward a more positive, nurturing relationship with your body. In the upcoming sections, we'll explore practical strategies to further support this growth, ensuring that your wellness journey is not only sustainable but also profoundly enriching.

Chapter 4

Nutrition and Fitness for Wellness: Nourishing Body and Mind

In our holistic journey to wellness, we now shift our focus to the vital components of nutrition and fitness.

This chapter explores the importance of science-backed nutrition for weight management, the incorporation of effective fitness strategies that support both our physical and emotional well-being, and the establishment

of a sustainable,
balanced routine.

Science-Backed Nutrition for Weight Management

Nutrition is the foundation of our physical and emotional well-being.

Science-backed nutrition offers a road map to support our weight management goals. We'll delve into the following key aspects:

Balanced Diet: The significance of consuming a variety of foods that provide essential nutrients.

Portion Control: Understanding appropriate portion sizes and strategies for mindful eating.

Caloric Awareness: Becoming conscious

of caloric intake and expenditure, all while maintaining a balanced approach.

Effective Fitness Strategies that Support Both Weight Management and Body Confidence

Fitness is not only a tool for weight management but a gateway to body confidence and mental well-being. We'll explore the following:

Diverse Exercise Modalities: The importance of incorporating various forms of exercise, including strength training, cardiovascular activities, and flexibility routines.

Mindful Movement: The power of mindful

exercise, where we connect with our bodies and focus on the present moment.

Progressive Overload: The concept of gradually increasing the intensity of workouts to facilitate growth and avoid plateaus.

Building a Sustainable, Balanced Routine

A sustainable, balanced routine is the cornerstone of our wellness journey. We'll discuss the following components:

Routine Variability:
How to infuse variety into your fitness routine to prevent boredom and burnout.

Periodization:
Structuring workouts in cycles to promote continual progress.

Rest and Recovery:
The necessity of
adequate rest and
recovery for physical
and mental well-being.

Incorporating science-
backed nutrition and
effective fitness
strategies into a

sustainable, balanced routine provides the basis for achieving your wellness goals. This chapter invites you to cultivate a well-rounded approach to nutrition and fitness that supports both weight management and body confidence. As we continue to explore the holistic path to wellness, you'll find practical strategies and guidance that enable you to apply these principles to your daily life, nurturing both your body and mind.

Chapter 5

Mindful Wellness: Nurturing Body and Mind

In our pursuit of holistic wellness, we now turn our attention to the powerful components of mindfulness and self-care. This chapter explores the role of mindfulness and self-care in weight management and body image, guides you on managing stress and building resilience, and emphasizes the importance of cultivating mental and emotional balance.

The Role of Mindfulness and Self-Care in Weight Management and Body Image

Mindfulness and self-care are essential

tools on our path to holistic wellness. We'll delve into their significance and application:

Mindful Eating: The practice of being present and fully engaged during meals, allowing us to savor our food, recognize hunger and fullness cues, and reduce emotional eating.

Self-Care Rituals: The nurturing practices that rejuvenate body and mind, fostering self-compassion, and supporting a positive body image.

Managing Stress and Building Resilience

Stress can be a significant obstacle on our wellness journey. In this section, we'll explore strategies for effectively managing stress and building resilience:

Stress Awareness: Recognizing the sources and symptoms of stress in your life.

Stress Management Techniques: Practical tools to reduce and cope with stress, including deep breathing, mindfulness meditation, and progressive muscle relaxation.

Building Resilience: Strengthening your emotional resilience to navigate life's challenges with grace and poise.

Cultivating Mental and Emotional Balance

Mental and emotional balance is at the core of our holistic wellness. We'll explore how to achieve this balance through:

Emotional Awareness: Recognizing and

processing your emotions in a healthy way.

Cognitive Reframing: Techniques to shift your thought patterns from negative to positive.

Mind-Body Connection: Understanding the profound link between your physical and mental health.

Mindful wellness is the glue that holds our holistic wellness journey together. By practicing mindfulness, self-care, managing stress, and cultivating mental and emotional balance, we strengthen our capacity to navigate challenges and appreciate the beauty of the present moment. As we continue to explore the holistic approach to wellness, you'll discover practical strategies to apply these principles to your daily life, nurturing both your body and mind.

Chapter 6

Building a Supportive Environment: The Foundation of Wellness

In our holistic journey to wellness, we recognize the critical importance of the environment in which we operate. This chapter focuses on the significance of creating a nurturing and supportive environment for your wellness goals, seeking social support and understanding, and navigating the pressures that society

may impose upon
your journey.

**Creating a Nurturing
and Supportive
Environment for Your
Wellness Goals**

A nurturing
environment is the
fertile soil in which

your wellness goals can thrive. We'll discuss strategies for creating this space, including:

Physical Environment: Organizing your surroundings to support your well-being, such as setting up a workout area at home or decluttering your living space.

Social Environment: Surrounding yourself with individuals who understand and support your wellness journey.

Seeking Social Support and Understanding

Support from friends and loved ones can significantly impact your journey. In this section, we explore the role of social support and understanding, including:

The Power of Community: The importance of finding like-minded individuals or support groups to connect with.

Effective Communication: Strategies for communicating your wellness goals and needs to those around you.

Setting Boundaries: Maintaining healthy

boundaries to protect your well-being.

Navigating Societal Pressures

Society can exert significant pressures on individuals striving for wellness. We'll discuss strategies for navigating these pressures, such as:

Resisting Unrealistic Standards: Recognizing and rejecting societal ideals that may not align with your own wellness goals.

Positive Self-Talk:
Techniques for countering negative self-talk that may arise from societal pressures.

Empowering Individuality: Embracing your unique journey and understanding that there's no one-size-fits-all approach to wellness.

Creating a nurturing environment, seeking support, and navigating societal pressures are essential components

of our holistic
approach to wellness.
By understanding the
power of your
environment, building
a support network,
and recognizing the
impact of societal
influences, you
empower yourself to
thrive on your unique
path to well-being. As

we continue to explore the holistic path to wellness, you'll discover practical strategies to apply these principles to your daily life, fostering a space in which your wellness goals are not only achievable but profoundly enriching.